Ketogenic Diet

Lose Over 15 lbs Fast & Easy
with Ketogenic Diet Full Plan!

Table of contents

Introduction

I would like to thank and congratulate you for downloading **"Ketogenic Diet: Lose over 15 lbs Fast & Easy Right Now with Ketogenic Diet Full Plan!"** Making the choice to go onto the ketogenic diet shows me that you are a person that wants to make changes in your lifestyle to help improve your health and well-being. This is a great diet choice especially for those that are very concerned about developing diabetes or have type two diabetes.

The ketogenic diet is basically low-carb and high in fats. When our primary source of calories are coming from the fat stored in our bodies ketones are formed. When the body is in ketosis it has higher levels of ketones in the blood. When our body is in a ketogenic state the bodies lipid energy metabolic is intact.

What the ketogenic diet is going to do is to help increase your bodies ability to make use of stored fats for fuel. When your body is no longer receiving high-carbohydrates it is then forced to become efficient in using stored fats as an energy source.

Another benefit of being in ketosis is that is has protein-sparing effects, assuming that you are already eating plenty of calories per day. Once your body is in ketosis it will prefer ketones over glucose.

If you want this diet to really work for you, then you need to be prepared to make a solid commitment to it and not cheat on this diet. In order for you to be satiated or full you need to make sure your are eating what is needed to achieve this. Remember that ketosis is a process that happens within your body, it takes time so sticking to the diet is important to get the proper effects. If you are not ready to make the full commitment to the diet it will not work. If you are ready to make this commitment, then I hope the recipes and meal planner I have provided will help your journey to better health be a more pleasant experience—good luck!

Chapter 1 – Starting a Ketogenic Diet

Beginning the ketogenic diet may involve getting some food supplies that you normally don't have in your kitchen cupboards such as milled flaxseed meal, Stevia, almond flour, and coconut flour. You may have to go to your local health food store for some of your supplies.

During the first week of the diet plan it is simple and easy to follow so that it will be and easier process for you in just starting out on a low carb diet. We don't want the transition to be a torturous one for you, when you begin to have cravings for carbs. In some of the recipes you are going to have leftovers so you can freeze them and have them at a later date, this will help save time by cooking one less meal. It certainly will come in handy when you are coming home from a long day at work and don't feel like do any cooking.

Ketosis is commonly referred to as the "keto flu" you may experience brain fogginess, headaches, and fatigue. During this process it is very important that you keep drinking plenty of water and eating salt. While you are on the ketogenic diet you are going to be peeing much more than you normally do. The reason for this is because it is a diuretic. During this time electrolytes are removed from your body. You need to make sure you are replacing your water and salt supply to keep your body hydrated and re-supply electrolytes. By making sure to do this you can avoid headaches. Try sprinkling some salt into your water that you are drinking. Keep taking some salt and make sure to drink at least four liters of water a day.

You may want to prepare. foods on weekend for your breakfasts for the week. This way you don't have to prepare them in the morning before going off to work. During the first week of lunches they will consist of meat and salad served with high fat dressing. You can use leftover meat from dinners for the next days lunch. You can add spices to your salads but not too much of garlic powders, or onion. Your dinners will consist of more veggies and meat, that will have moderate protein and high on good fats. There is no deserts included in the first two weeks of a ketogenic diet.

The best thing to do before you go shopping is to make a grocery list for the items you will need to make your first week of meals. Then when you go shopping stick to the items on your list. If an item is not on the list then you shouldn't be buying it. Avoid going into aisles that are full of junk foods filled with high amounts of carbs—these are foods that you must avoid while on the ketogenic diet plan.

Another good idea when starting any kind of diet plan is to inform your friends and loved ones that you are going on a diet and ask them not to encourage you to go off your diet by offering you foods you should not be eating. Most people will be very understanding and will make an effort to support you while you are trying to stick to your diet. If they are made aware of when you are starting your diet they are not going to show up at your door with a box of doughnuts. Sometimes it is good to have some kind of support system in play when you are going on a diet. There is websites that have other people that are dieting too that help give each other support during those tough times during the process of dieting.

You may want to consider going on the diet plan with another such as a family member or friend. You can then help each other stick to the diet plan by offering each other support and encouragement. When going through challenges in life such as diets it is always a good idea to have a support system in place. We all need encouragement to help us over those tough hurdles we will face in life's challenges. Our support system can remind us what our goal is and why we are on the diet in the first place. This will help remind us that we are going to benefit greatly by sticking to the diet, even when at times it feels like we don't think we can make it to the end. It is amazing what a little bit of support and encouragement can do for us when we need it most.

Chapter 2 – Ketogenic Diet Meal Planner

Day 1

Breakfast

Frittata Muffins (two muffins)

Per Serving

Calories: 410

Fats: 32.3g

Net Carbs: 2.5g

Protein: 27.3g

Lunch

Spinach Salad

Per Serving

Calories: 537

Fats: 57g

Net Carbs: 1g

Dinner

Sausage & Chicken Stir-fry

Freeze leftovers for two more meals, add a quarter of a cup of shredded cheddar to meal not to leftovers.

Per Serving

Calories: 541

Fats: 8.3g

Net Carbs: 8.3g

Protein: 42.7g

Day 2

Breakfast

Scrambled Eggs with Cheese

Per Serving

Calories: 453

Fats: 43g

Net Carbs: 1.2g

Protein: 19g

Lunch

Canned Chicken & Spinach Salad

Per Serving

Calories: 450

Fats: 44g

Net Carbs: 0.5g

Protein: 13.5g

Dinner

Bacon Burger & Red Pepper Salad

Per Serving

Calories: 641

Fats: 52.5g

Net Carbs: 4.7g

Protein: 37g

Day 3

Breakfast

Frittata Muffins (two muffins)

Per Serving

Calories: 410

Fats: 32.3g

Net Carbs: 2.5g

Protein: 27.3g

Lunch

Leftover Bacon Burger & Spinach Salad

Per Serving

Calories: 624

Fats: 63.9g

Net Carbs: 1.2g

Protein: 10.8g

Dinner

Cinnamon & Orange Beef Stew

Per Serving

Calories: 519

Fats: 35.6g

Net Carbs: 4.1g

Protein: 42.8g

Day 4

Breakfast

Scrambled Eggs with Cheese

Per Serving

Calories: 453

Fats: 43g

Net Carbs: 1.2g

Protein: 19g

Lunch

Leftover Cinnamon & Orange Stew

Per Serving

Calories: 519

Fats: 35.6g

Net Carbs: 4.1g

Protein: 42.8g

Dinner

Cauliflower & Shrimp Curry

Eat one sixth of recipe and freeze the rest as five portions.

Per Serving

Calories: 451

Fats: 33.5g

Net Carbs: 5.6g

Protein: 27.4g

Day 5

Breakfast

Frittata Muffins (two muffins)

Per Serving

Calories: 410

Fats: 32.3g

Net Carbs: 2.5g

Protein: 27.3g

Lunch

Leftover Cauliflower & Shrimp Curry

Per Serving

Calories: 451

Fats: 33.5g

Net Carbs: 5.6g

Protein: 27.4g

Dinner

Chorizo & Cheddar Meatballs & Roasted Pecan Green Beans

Freeze the leftovers

Per Serving

Calories: 798

Fats: 63g

Net Carbs: 7.1g

Protein: 40.2g

Day 6

Breakfast

Scrambled Eggs with Cheese

Per Serving

Calories: 453

Fats: 43g

Net Carbs: 1.2g

Protein: 19g

Lunch

Spinach Salad with Cream Cheese

Per Serving

Calories: 496

Fats: 51g

Net Carbs: 2g

Proteins: 5g

Dinner

Curry Chicken Thigh with Fried Queso Fresco

Per Serving

Calories: 657

Fats: 44.7g

Net Carbs: 0.6g

Protein: 40.3g

Day 7

Breakfast

Scrambled Eggs with Cheese

Per Serving

Calories: 553

Fats: 55g

Net Carbs: 1.2g

Protein: 19g

Lunch

Leftover Curry Chicken & Spinach Salad

Per Serving

Calories: 586

Fats: 58g

Net Carbs: 1g

Protein: 15g

Dinner

Chili & Sugar Snap Peas

Eat one quarter of total recipe then freeze leftovers that will leave you with three more portions.

Per Serving

Calories: 545

Fats: 31.1g

Net Carbs: 9.6g

Proteins: 53.1g

Chapter 3 – Week 2 of Ketogenic Diet

You have made it through the first week of the ketogenic diet congrads to you, I hope that you found it fairly easy to stick with and follow the meal plan. At this point in the diet we are adding "Bulletproof Coffee" into the menu. This is a great tasting coffee made from a blend of coconut milk, grass-fed butter, and heavy cream. You might be thinking what a strange recipe for coffee, but when you taste this rich and decadent tasting coffee I am sure you are going to enjoy this new addition to the menu.

If you are not a person that drinks coffee you can also add this to your tea. The bullet proof coffee is great at helping with fat loss. In the bulletproof coffee you will be taking in medium-chain triglycerides or MCT's that have been shown to lead to greater loses of fat tissue, in both animals and humans. By eating these fats you are going to have more efficient energy usage, along with better results in your overall weight loss.

What medium-chain fatty acids or MCFAs lead to are an increase in energy expenditure, they are converted into ketones, which are absorbed differently by your body compared to other oils, giving you a much better overall energy. You can also add spices and sweeteners to this if you like. I like to add some cinnamon to mine.

With your second week lunches continue to use the leftovers from the previous nights dinner along with a nice green salad topped with some high fat dressing. Through the proper use of this diet plan it will help you to lose the weight that you want in a healthy way. Remember there is to be no deserts in the first two weeks of the ketogenic diet.

Focus on your goals that you hope to reach by using the ketogenic diet, and make sure to stick with your diet and before you know you will be finishing it feeling and looking better than you have in a very long time! Keep up the good work and good luck with your second week—you can do it!

Day 8

Breakfast

Bulletproof Coffee

Per Serving

Calories: 273g

Fats: 30g

Net Carbs: 1g

Protein: 0g

Lunch

Cheddar, Chive, & Bacon Cake

Per Serving

Calories: 573

Fats: 55g

Net Carbs: 5g

Proteins: 24g

Dinner

Leftover Chorizo Meatballs and Roasted Pecan Green Beans

Per Serving

Calories: 921

Fats: 72.2g

Net Carbs: 7.9g

Protein: 47.5g

Day 9

Breakfast

Bulletproof Coffee

Per Serving.

Calories: 273

Fats: 30g

Net Carbs: 1g

Protein: 0g

Lunch

Taco Tartlets (eat two for one serving)

Per Serving.

Calories: 481

Fats: 38.8g

Net Carbs: 5.47g

Protein: 26.2g

Dinner

Buffalo Chicken Strips (refrigerate two strips, eat one third of the recipe and freeze the rest of leftovers)

Sugar Snap Peas (one portion)

Per Serving.

Calories: 750 calories

Fats: 58.7g

Net Carbs: 9.1g

Protein: 42.3g

Day 10

Breakfast

Bulletproof Coffee

Per Serving.

Calories: 273

Fats: 30g

Net Carbs: 1g

Protein: 0g

Lunch

Leftover Chicken Strips on Almond Bun

Per Serving.

Calories: 625

Fats: 51g

Net Carbs: 5.3g

Proteins: 49.1g

Dinner

Bacon Mozzarella Meatballs (five meatballs freeze leftovers)

Roasted Pecan Green Beans (Eat one portion use leftovers)

Per Serving.

Calories: 821

Fats: 63.8g

Net Carbs: 6.7g

Protein: 54g

Day 11

Breakfast

Bulletproof Coffee

Per Serving

Calories: 273

Fats: 30g

Net Carbs: 1g

Protein: 0g

Lunch

Leftover Burger& Spinach Salad

Per Serving

Calories: 510

Fats: 42g

Net Carbs: 2.4g

Protein: 25.9g

Dinner

Burger with Creamed Spinach & Almonds (eat half of the total recipe and refrigerate leftovers)

Almond Flax Bun add one tablespoon of butter to bun.

Per Serving.

Calories: 773

Fats: 59.9g

Net Carbs: 5.3g

Proteins: 49.1g

Day 12

Breakfast

Bulletproof Coffee

Per Serving

Calories: 273

Fats: 30g

Net Carbs: 1g

Protein: 0g

Lunch

Leftover Tartlets (Eat two)

Per Serving

Calories: 481

Fats: 38.8g

Net Carbs: 4.8g

Protein: 50.3g

Dinner

Chicken Sausage Stir Fry Leftovers (add one quarter cup of cheese and one tablespoon of butter)

Per Serving.

Calories: 641

Fats: 49.3g

Net Carbs: 8.3g

Protein: 42.7g

Day 13

Breakfast

Bulletproof Coffee

Per Serving.

Calories: 273

Fats: 30g

Net Carbs: 1g

Protein: 0g

Lunch

Leftover Mozzarella Meatballs & Spinach Salad

Per Serving

Calories: 641

Fats: 51.2g

Net Carbs: 3g

Protein: 35.2g

Dinner

Leftover Chili served with sugar snap peas

Per Serving

Calories: 545

Fats: 31.1g

Net Carbs: 9.6g

Protein: 53.1g

Day 14

Breakfast

Bulletproof Coffee

Per Serving

Calories: 273

Fats: 30g

Net Carbs: 1g

Proteins: 0g

Lunch

Chive, Cheddar & Bacon Mug Cake

Per Serving

Calories: 573

Fats: 55g

Net Carbs: 5g

Proteins: 24g

Dinner

Leftover Cauliflower & Shrimp Curry (use one tablespoon of extra butter and double serving)

Per Serving

Calories: 661

Fats: 39g

Net Carbs: 11.2g

Protein: 54.8g

Chapter 4- Recipes 1-15 of Ketogenic Meal Planner

1. Chili

Ingredients:

- two pounds of beef stew meat
- one third cup of tomato paste
- one green pepper
- one cup of beef broth
- two tablespoons of chili powder
- two tablespoons of soy sauce
- two tablespoons of coconut oil
- one yellow onion

Directions:

Divide your stew meat making half of it into small cubes, the other half put into food processor and make ground beef. Next chop onion and pepper up into small pieces. Add spices with sauce. Saute the cubed stew beef in pan over medium heat in coconut oil until browned, then transfer to slow-cooker. Do the same process with your ground beef. Saute the veggies in the remaining fat for a few minutes. Now add all ingredients to slow-cooker and mix well. Cook on high for two and a half hours then switch to low and cook for another half hour with the lid off.

2. Sugar Snap Peas

Ingredients:

- two teaspoons of garlic, minced
- three cups of sugar snap peas
- juice of half a lemon
- half a teaspoon of red pepper flakes

Directions:

In a pan add three tablespoons of bacon fat over medium heat, add garlic, and reduce the heat for one minute. Then add the sugar peas and lemon juice and cook for another few minutes. Remove from heat put onto serving dish garnish with red pepper flakes and lemon zest.

3. Roasted Pecan Green Beans

Ingredients:

half a teaspoon of red pepper flakes

- *half a pound of green beans*
- *two tablespoons of Parmesan cheese*
- *one quarter of a cup of pecans, chopped*
- *two tablespoons of olive oil*
- *half a lemon's zest*
- *one teaspoon of garlic, minced*

Directions:

Preheat your oven to 450 then add your pecans to food processor. Then grind the pecans in the food processor until they are chopped. There should be some small and large pieces. In mixing bowl mix with green beans, olive oil, Parmesan cheese, lemon zest, minced garlic, and red pepper flakes. Spread out the green beans on a foiled baking sheet. Roast beans for twenty-five minutes. Allow beans to cool for five minutes then serve!

4. Cream Cheese & Spinach Salad

Ingredients:

- *four cups of spinach*
- *three tablespoons of olive oil*
- *one ounce of cream cheese*

Directions:

Wash your spinach, then dry with paper towel to get rid of the excess water, chop, and put into salad bowl. Then add three tablespoons of olive oil and one ounce of cream cheese and lightly toss and serve.

5. Chorizo & Cheddar Meatballs

Ingredients:

- *one cup of cheddar cheese*
- *two Chorizo sausages*
- *two large eggs*
- *one third of a cup of crushed pork rinds*
- *one cup of tomato sauce, low-carb*
- *one teaspoon of chili powder*
- *one teaspoon of cumin*
- *one and a half pounds of ground beef*
- *one tablespoon of salt*

Directions:

Preheat your oven to 350 degrees Fahrenheit. Now take your sausage and break it up into small pieces and then mix with ground beef, ground pork rinds, cheese, spices, and eggs. Make sure to mix well, then form meatballs place these on a baking tray lined with foil. Bake for 35 minutes or until the meatballs are cooked through. Spoon tomato sauce over meatball and serve.

6. Curry Chicken Thigh

Ingredients for chicken thighs:

- *one eighth teaspoon of allspice*

- *half a teaspoon of yellow curry*

- *one quarter teaspoon of paprika*

- *half a teaspoon of salt*

- *pinch of cinnamon*

- *one tablespoon of olive oil*

- *two chicken thighs*

- *pinch of ginger*

- *one eighth teaspoon of coriander*

- *one eighth teaspoon of chili*

- *one quarter teaspoon of garlic powder*

- *one eighth of a teaspoon of cayenne pepper*

Directions:

Preheat your oven to 425 degrees Fahrenheit. Then mix all of your spices in a bowl. Cover a baking sheet in foil then place the chicken thighs onto it. Rub olive oil over the thighs evenly. Rub spice mixture on both sides of chicken thighs. Bake for 50 minutes. Let cool for five minutes before serving them and enjoy!

Ingredients for Queso Fresco:

- *one pound of Queso Fresco or Paneer cheese*
- *one tablespoon of coconut oil*
- *half a tablespoon of olive oil*

Directions:

First you will want to cut your cheese into cubes or thin rectangles. Heat one tablespoon of coconut oil and half a tablespoon of olive oil over high heat then add cheese. Allow it cook until it is browned on one side then flip over and brown the other side. Remove it from pan drain excess grease on paper towel.

7. Shrimp & Cauliflower Curry

Ingredients:

- *four cups of chicken stock*
- *one cup of coconut milk*
- *five cups of raw spinach*
- *one medium onion*
- *one quarter cup of heavy cream*
- *twenty-four ounces of shrimp, deveined, and peeled*
- *half a head of medium cauliflower*
- *one quarter cup of butter*

- *three tablespoons of olive oil*

- *one teaspoon of onion powder*

- *one fourth a teaspoon of cardamom*

- *half a teaspoon of Turmeric*

- *half a teaspoon of coriander*

- *half a teaspoon of ginger*

- *one teaspoon of paprika*

- *one teaspoon of cayenne*

- *one tablespoon of coconut flour*

- *one teaspoon of chili powder*

- *two teaspoons of garlic powder*

- *one fourth a teaspoon of cinnamon*

- *two tablespoons of curry powder*

- *one tablespoon of cumin*

- *one fourth a teaspoon of Xanthan gum*

Directions:

Take all of your spices except for coconut flour and xanthan gum set these aside. Cut up your onion into slices. In pan heat olive oil over medium heat add onion slices, cook until they are soft. Then add your butter, heavy cream and one eighth of a teaspoon of xanthan gum and spices making sure to mix well. After two minutes add four cups of chicken broth, and one cup of coconut milk. Make sure to stir well and cover. Cook for 30 minutes with lid on. Chop up cauliflower into small florets then add your curry at this point. Cook for another fifteen minutes covered. Now add shrimp into curry. Cook for an additional twenty minutes with the lid off. Add your coconut flour and one eighth teaspoon of xanthan gum and stir well. Cook for another ten minutes with the lid off.

8. Cinnamon & Orange Beef Stew

Ingredients:

- *three quarter cup of Beef broth*
- *half a teaspoon of cinnamon, ground*
- *three quarter of a teaspoon of Thyme*
- *zest of of orange*
- *one quarter of yellow onion*
- *one tablespoon of coconut oil*
- *one quarter teaspoon of sage*
- *one quarter pound of ground beef*
- *half a teaspoon of fish sauce*
- *one bay leaf*
- *one quarter cup of orange juice*
- *one quarter teaspoon of rosemary*
- *half a teaspoon of Soy sauce*

Directions:

Dice your veggies and cut your meat into one inch cubes. Zest a whole orange. Now heat your coconut oil in a skillet, then add salt, pepper, and meat to skillet in batches. Do not over fill your skillet. When you have finished browning your meat remove meat from pan and add vegetables to pan cooking for two minutes. Then add orange juice to pan and other ingredients except for sage, rosemary and thyme. Allow to cook for a moment then transfer all ingredients to your crock pot. Cook for three hours on high. Now your crockpot add the rest of your spices to the pot. Cook for one to two hours on high then enjoy!

9. Spinach Salad

Ingredients:

- add seasonings of your choice
- four tablespoons of olive oil
- four cups of spinach

Directions:

Wash your spinach then pat dry with paper towel to remove excess water from your spinach. Now chop spinach into desired size. Add olive oil and spinach in salad bowl adding seasoning of your choice toss lightly and serve.

10. Chicken Sausage Stir Fry

Ingredients:

- half a cup of tomato sauce low-carb
- two tablespoons of salted butter
- one quarter cup of red wine
- three cups of broccoli florets
- half a cup of Parmesan cheese
- three cups of spinach
- four chicken sausages
- half a teaspoon of red pepper flakes
- two teaspoons of garlic, minced

Directions:

Start to boil a pot of water on the stove, and slice up your sausage. Then add your sausages to a pan on high heat. Put your broccoli into the boiling water and cook for five minutes. Stir your sausages around in pan until they brown on both sides. Move sausages to one side of pan then add the butter. Place garlic in the butter and saute for one minute. Then mix everything together, adding the broccoli. Pour your tomato sauce, red wine, and red pepper flakes over. Mix together, add your spinach with salt and pepper and let cook on simmer for ten minutes. Finally add Parmesan cheese to the top before serving.

11. Canned Chicken & Spinach Salad

Ingredients:

- *one can of chicken or can use other canned meats such as turkey, or ham*

- *two tablespoons of Parmesan cheese*

- *one quarter of Lemon zest*

- *two cups of spinach*

- *four tablespoons of olive oil*

- *one and a half teaspoons of Dijon mustard*

- *three quarters of a teaspoon of curry powder, optional*

Directions:

Mix all of your wet ingredients in a bowl. Mix together your meat and spinach in a bowl. Pour the wet ingredients into bowl with meat in it when you are ready to eat it.

12. Frittata Muffins

Ingredients:

- *eight large eggs*
- *half a teaspoon of pepper*
- *half a cup of cheddar cheese*
- *one tablespoon of butter*
- *four ounces of bacon, precooked and chopped*
- *half a cup of half and half cream*
- *two teaspoons of Parsley, dried*
- *one quarter teaspoon of salt*

Directions:

Preheat the oven to 375 degrees Fahrenheit. Mix eggs with the half and half in a bowl. Add bacon and cheese, as well as spices. Add any other additional ingredients at this point. Grease the muffin tray with butter. You will yield eight muffins from this recipe. Pour the mixture into each muffin cup filling three quarters full. Put into oven for 20 minutes or until they are golden and puffy on the edges. Remove muffins from oven allow to cool for one minute. You can freeze these and heat individually.

13. Bacon Burger and Red Pepper Salad

Ingredients for Burger:

- *200g of ground beef*
- *one and a half teaspoons of Chives, chopped*
- *half a teaspoon of salt*
- *one quarter teaspoon of onion powder*
- *half a teaspoon of black pepper*
- *three quarter of a teaspoon of Soy sauce*
- *two tablespoons of Cheddar cheese*
- *two slices of bacon, chopped*
- *half a teaspoon of garlic, minced*
- *one quarter of a teaspoon of Worcestershire*

Ingredients for Red pepper salad:

- *two tablespoons of Ranch dressing*
- *one and a half tablespoons of Parmesan*
- *three cups of spinach*
- *half a teaspoon of red pepper flakes*

Directions:

In your skillet cook your chopped bacon until it is nice and crisp. Then remove it from pan and place on paper towel. Drain your grease and save it. In a mixing bowl combine chopped bacon, spices, and ground beef. Form into three patties. In your pan put two tablespoons of bacon fat. Once your bacon fat is heated place patties into pan. Cook for five minutes on each side of your patties. Then remove from pan let rest for five minutes. Serve with cheese, and extra bacon, and onion if this would suit your taste.

14. Scrambled Eggs with Cheese

Ingredients:

- *one teaspoon of Chive, chopped*
- *two large eggs*
- *add spices of your choice*
- *two tablespoons of butter*
- *one ounce of cheddar, shredded*

Directions:

Heat your frying pan on stove over medium heat, then add butter. Once your butter has melted add your eggs to the pan. Scramble eggs before adding to pan. Let the eggs cook on low heat. Then add your seasonings, chives, salt, pepper, hot sauce if you want it to taste more spicy or hot. Add the shredded cheese and mix together.

15. Cheddar, Bacon, & Chive Cake

Ingredients:

- *two tablespoons of white cheddar, shredded*
- *two tablespoons of almond flour*
- *two slices of bacon*
- *two tablespoons of butter*
- *one egg*
- *half a teaspoon of baking powder*
- *one tablespoon of Chives, chopped*
- *pinch of salt*
- *one quarter of a teaspoon of Mrs. Dash*
- *one tablespoon of cheddar cheese, shredded*

Directions:

Take all of your ingredients and mix in microwaveable stoneware bowl. Then spray inside of bowl with non-stick cooking spray. Microwave for 70 seconds. Remove from micro and turn upside down lightly bang against plate.

Chapter 5 – Recipes 16-24 of Ketogenic Recipes

16. BBQ Pulled Chicken

Makes 4 Servings

Ingredients:

- *one quarter of a cup of red wine*
- *two tablespoons of spicy brown mustard*
- *one teaspoon of cumin*
- *two teaspoons of chili powder*
- *one tablespoon of Soy sauce*
- *one tablespoon of liquid smoke*
- *two tablespoons of spicy brown mustard*
- *six chicken thighs, boneless, skinless*
- *one quarter cup of organic tomato paste*
- *one quarter of a cup of chicken stock*
- *one quarter cup of Stevia*
- *one third of a cup of salted butter*
- *one teaspoon of cayenne pepper*

Directions:

Mix all of your ingredients except for chicken thighs. Put chicken thighs into slow cooker and pour sauce over them. Cook on low for eight hours. Take chicken and shred it down, for this you can use two forks. Mix around your sauce and cook for an additional 45 minutes on high.

17. Ginger Beef

Makes two servings

Ingredients:

- *four tablespoons of apple cider vinegar*
- *two sirloin steaks*
- *one teaspoon of ginger, ground*
- *salt and pepper to taste*
- *two small diced tomatoes*
- *one clove of garlic, crushed*
- *one tablespoon of olive oil*
- *one small diced yellow onion*

Directions:

Put your oil into a large skillet over medium heat, once oil is hot add steaks, brown them. Add to the pan your garlic, onion, and tomatoes once both sides of steak are browned. Then cover the skillet and maintain low heat. Let simmer until all liquids have evaporated from your pan.

18.   Keto Cookies

Makes 14 cookies

Ingredients:

- two cups of almond flour
- one tablespoon of Stevia
- one tablespoon of vanilla
- one quarter cup of sugar-free Maple syrup
- one quarter cup of coconut oil
- two cups of almond flour
- one quarter of a teaspoon of baking soda
- two tablespoons of cinnamon

Directions:

Preheat your oven to 350 degrees Fahrenheit. In a bowl mix your baking soda, almond flour, and salt. In another bowl mix maple syrup, coconut oil, vanilla, and Stevia. Mix your dry ingredients into your wet ingredients mix until dough is formed. Mix your cinnamon and Erythritol together until a powder is formed. Roll the dough into balls. Roll them into the cinnamon mixture, set them on baking tray that has been sprayed with non-stick cooking spray. Then flatten the balls and put into oven and bake for ten minutes, remove and let cool.

19. Spicy Cakes

Makes 10 cakes

Ingredients for cake mix

- *half a teaspoon of cinnamon*
- *one teaspoon of vanilla*
- *two teaspoons of baking powder*
- *four large eggs*
- *half a teaspoon of allspice*
- *three quarter cup of Erythritol*
- *two cups of almond flour*
- *one quarter teaspoon of clove, ground*
- *half a teaspoon of ginger*
- *half a teaspoon of nutmeg*
- *five tablespoons of water*
- *half a cup of salted butter*

Ingredients for Cream Cheese Frosting:

- *one teaspoon of vanilla extract*
- *two tablespoons of butter*
- *eight ounces of cream cheese*
- *zest of half a lemon*
- *three tablespoons of Erythritol*

Directions:

Preheat your oven to 350 degrees Fahrenheit. In a mixing bowl add sweetener and butter. Cream them together until they are smooth. Add two eggs and continue to mix. Add last two eggs. Grind up your spices using a pestle and mortar then add to batter. Mix until smooth. Add the water and mix until it is creamy. Spray cupcake tray with non-stick cooking spray. Fill cups up with batter three quarter of the way. Place in the oven for 15 minutes. While they are baking cream together your cream cheese and your butter, sweetener, vanilla, lemon zest to make frosting. Remove the cupcakes from oven allow them to cool for 15 minutes then frost them.

20. Veggie Delight

Makes 3 Servings

Ingredients:

- one teaspoon of pepper
- one teaspoon of salt
- two teaspoons of garlic, minced
- two tablespoons of pumpkin seeds
- 90g of spinach
- 90g of bell pepper, yellow
- 100g of sugar snap peas
- 115g of broccoli
- half a teaspoon of red pepper flakes
- six tablespoons of extra virgin olive oil
- 240g of baby Bella mushrooms

Directions:

Chop up all of your veggies into small bite size pieces. Then heat the oil adding garlic and saute for one minute, now add mushrooms and allow them to soak up the oil. Next add broccoli and mix well. Allow the broccoli to cook for a few minutes, then, add your sugar snap peas. Then throw in your bell peppers, and pumpkin seeds. Once cooked lay spinach on top until it is wilted, mix and serve.

21. Vanilla Cookies

Makes 10 cookies

Ingredients:

half a teaspoon of salt

- half a teaspoon of baking soda
- one tablespoon + one teaspoon of instant coffee grounds
- two large eggs
- 15 drops of liquid Stevia
- half a cup of unsalted butter
- one and a half cups of almond flour
- one third a cup of Erythritol
- one quarter of a teaspoon of cinnamon
- one and a half teaspoons of vanilla

Directions:

Preheat your oven to 350 degrees Fahrenheit. Mix in a bowl, cinnamon, coffee grounds, almond flour, salt and baking soda. In another bowl separate whites and egg yolks. In another mixing bowl add butter and beat adding Erythritol to butter and continue to beat until it is almost white. Then add your egg yolks to the butter mix blend until smooth. Take half of the mixed almond flour and add to the butter and mix. Add vanilla extract and liquid Stevia, add the rest of almond mix. Mix well to combine. Beat your egg whites until they are stiff, fold them into the cookie dough. Divide your cookies on a cookie sheet and make ten large cookies. Bake them for 15 minutes. Remove from oven to cooling rack allowing to cool for 15 minutes.

22. Bacon Wrapped Pork Tenderloin

Makes one serving with leftovers

Ingredients:

- half a pound of pork tenderloin
- pinch of black pepper
- one quarter of a teaspoon of rosemary, dried
- one quarter of a teaspoon of liquid smoke
- one quarter of a teaspoon of garlic, minced
- three quarter of a teaspoon of Soy sauce
- one and a half teaspoon of sugar-free Maple syrup
- one and a half teaspoons of Dijon mustard
- three slices of bacon
- pinch of cayenne

Directions:

Add all of the wet ingredients together and dry ingredients to make a marinade. Dry pat your pork tenderloin with a paper towel then add to a zip-lock bag. Add the marinade into bag, rub marinade into meat. Place into fridge for five hours.

Preheat your oven to 350 degrees Fahrenheit. Place pork on piece of foil and wrap in bacon. Bake for one hour, then broil for ten minutes. Cover the tenderloin with foil for ten minutes to rest. Serve and enjoy!

24. Keto Cookies

Makes 14 cookies

Ingredients:

- *two tablespoons of cinnamon*
- *one quarter cup of sugar-free Maple syrup*
- *one quarter cup of coconut oil*
- *two cups of almond flour*
- *one tablespoon of Stevia*
- *one quarter of a teaspoon of baking soda*
- *one tablespoon of vanilla*

Directions:

Preheat oven to 350 degrees Fahrenheit. Mix in a bowl your baking soda, almond flour, and salt. In a separate bowl mix maple syrup, coconut oil, vanilla, and Stevia. Mix the dry ingredients into the wet ingredients mix until dough is formed. Mix cinnamon and Erythritol together until a powder is formed. Roll the dough into balls. Roll them into the cinnamon mixture, set them on baking tray that has been sprayed with non-stick cooking spray. Flatten the balls then put into oven and bake for ten minutes, remove and let cool.

25. Meatloaf

Makes 6 servings

Ingredients:

- two tablespoons of barbecue sauce
- one quarter cup of heavy cream
- half a teaspoon of black pepper, ground
- two teaspoons of Dijon mustard
- one quarter cup of parsley leaves
- one teaspoon of salt
- one teaspoon of basil, fresh, chopped
- one tablespoon of thyme leaves
- one cup of chopped green pepper
- two large eggs
- eight ounces of white onion, chopped
- five garlic cloves, minced
- eight ounces of cream cheese, softened
- two tablespoons of butter
- half a cup of shredded parmesan cheese
- two cups of shredded cheddar cheese
- half a cup of almond flour
- one pound of Italian sausage
- half a teaspoon of unflavored gelatin
- two pounds of ground beef

Directions:

Preheat the oven to 350 degrees Fahrenheit. Oil a baking dish with butter and put aside. Whisk the almond flour and parmesan cheese together in bowl, then set aside. Mix the cheddar cheese and softened cream cheese in another bowl until it has formed the texture of butter. In a skillet melt butter then add onion, garlic, and pepper. Let this cook for eight or so minutes until they are softened. Set aside and allow to cool.

Add your remaining ingredients in a food processor for a few seconds until the vegetables are minced. Blend eggs with salt, pepper, spices, barbecue sauce, mustard, and cream in another bowl. Add the gelatin on top and leave if for five minutes or so. Mix onion mixture and set aside. Mix the sausage and beef together. Add the meatloaf mixture back into the large mixing bowl adding egg mixture, mix well. Add the almond flour mixture combine well until the meat no longer sticks. Cover a cookie sheet with wax paper placing meat mixture on there to form a flat slab shape. Spread the slab with your cream cheese mixture. Take the meat and roll up covering the ends to protect the cheese mixture from spilling out. Let bake until browned for 30 minutes. Slice and serve and enjoy!

Conclusion

The ketogenic diet is fast becoming a popular choice of diet for many, and is certainly one healthy ways to quickly lose weight. The ketogenic diet was originally designed for people that have been battling with epilepsy. It is also beneficial for those that are looking to get their diabetes under control, that want to lose weight or for those looking for a healthier diet. I hope that you will find the meal planner and recipes helpful to you in your personal journey towards finding the perfect healthier lifestyle choice for yourself.

The ketogenic diet will help you will in achieving your goals for better health!

Thanks again for downloading my book if you have a moment I would greatly appreciate if you could leave a review for my book on Amazon, thanks and good luck with your new healthy eating habits!

www.ingramcontent.com/pod-product-compliance
Lightning Source LLC
Chambersburg PA
CBHW070449290526
45791CB00005B/2104